MACROS 101

Your Guide to Macros Calories Nutrition Labels Tracking & More

BONUSES INCLUDE:
MACROS FOOD OPTIONS LIST MALE/FEMALE MEAL PLAN
DETOX MEAL PLAN FAST FOOR OPTIONS LIST

by
Ellie Perico

Copyright © 2021 Ellie Perico
All Rights Reserved

TABLE OF CONTENTS

MACROS	1
MACROS FOOD LIST	4
Calculating Daily Calories	6
Calculating Daily Macros Needs	8
Sample Macros Ratios	13
My Fitness Pal	14
Reading Nutrition Labels	16
Macro Meal Plan - Female - 1200 to 1600	23
Macro Meal Plan - Male - 1700 - 2,000	40
Best Fast Food Options	60

MACROS

A topic that seems impossible to understand for so many but it's so much easier than it seems! Macros are the macronutrients that your body needs for growth and development. The 3 macros are Protein, Fats & Carbohydrates. Below is a graph to help explain each one with a visual. You'll see that some foods are made up of only one macronutrient (red, blue or green sections) while others have 2 or all 3 (white sections).

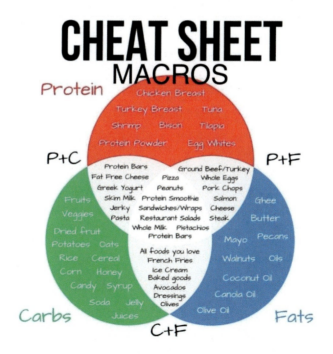

When you don't eat macros in the appropriate ratio for your goals, you don't see the results you want. You might be in a calorie deficit (eat less calories than your body burns each day) and you may still lose weight on the scale, but you won't see the results when it comes to leaning out and building muscle. These changes don't come until you combine a healthy diet, balanced macros AND effective workouts (if building muscle is one of your goals). This is when people get frustrated.

They say "I eat right & workout but I don't see results". Well that's because macros aren't balanced. You might be in your calorie range but you may not be getting enough protein, may be eating too many carbs and/or a combination of both. This is where tracking & understanding your macro ratio goals helps tremendously. And sometimes peoole THINK they're in a calorie deficit but they're not. Unless you're tracking and incorporating ALL of this (calorie deficit + macros balanced + workouts), you don't really know.

So, let's get to learning.
Click this LINK https://youtu.be/CmjTOoX5abU for a brief intro on macros. Then keep reading to calculate your macros using the info below & feel free to message me with any questions.

You can reach me via email at ellieperico@aol.com or send me a message on Instagram through my profile @fitcopmom. I'm always available for questions and am happy to connect with you and help you as a thank you for supporting me & purchasing my book. If you purchased the paperback and would like the links sent to you via email or message on IG, I can do that as well! Thank you again for the support and I hope you benefit from this book as much as I did when I learned what macros were & changed my life!

MACROS FOOD LIST

This next list in columns is a more detailed list version of the graphic above. It also includes both High Fiber AND Low Fiber carbs. High fiber carbs are always a better option but both can be part of a healthy diet. Use the list as a guide for ideas when it comes to making macro food choices. You can also print it out & use as a shopping list. Remember to try and stick to clean foods 80-90% of the time & the not so clean choices (candy, soda, dessert, cocktails, packaged/processed foods, foods high in sugar, etc) 10-20% of the time.

PROTEINS	CARBS	CARBS	FATS	FREEBIES
L= Lean HF = High fat	FFCs (High Fiber Carbs)	Low Fiber and/or High sugar Carb	Some Proteins are also fats	Foods You Can Have Unlimited
Egg Whites (L) Whey or Pea Protein Powder (L) Turkey Brest - ground or sliced (L) Extra Lean Ground Beef (96/4 or 98/2) (L) Lean cuts of beef (Inside Round, Sirloin) (L) Sushi grade or canned tuna (L) Low fat Cheese (L) Low fat Cottage Cheese (L) Low fat Greek Yogurt (L) Shrimp (L) Calamari (L) White Fish (L) Chicken Thighs (HF) Ground Beef 90/10, 80/20 (HF) Chicken Wings (HF) Salmon (HF)	Greens and lettuce Asparagus Zucchini Summer Squash Cauliflower Green Beans Peppers Mushrooms Tomatoes Spaghetti Squash Berries Melon Kiwi Citrus fruits (oranges, grapefruit, lemon, lime) Rice Cakes	Tropical Fruit (Mango, Papaya) Dried Fruit Bananas Flavored Yogurts Sweet/White Potato RIce Oatmeal (Gluten Free) Corn Tortillas English Muffins/Bread (Gluten Free) Cereal Pasta	All oils Coconut, grape seed & olive are best Avocado Nuts Nut Butters Whole Eggs Full Fat Dairy Salad Dressings Mayonnaise **Proteins w/ fat** ――――― Salmon Chicken other than breast Turkey other than breast All pork	-Mustards (Dijon, Stone Ground, Yellow) -Spices (Garlic Powder, Onion Powder, Salt, Pepper, Italian Seasoning, Lemon Pepper) -Hot Sauces (without added sugars) -Salsa -pick de gallo -Black coffee -unsweetened tea -Broth -fresh herbs -horseradish -And in my book, ALL leafy greens are freebies! I eat a LOT of spinach each day and don't count it much! Nobody ever got fat from eating leaves lol!

Calculating Daily Calories

Without a calorie deficit it's difficult to know how much you can & should eat each day to lose weight. So we have to do that calculation first, before calculating your macros needs.

Look at the photo below. This is very important & I've modified it from how I used to do it! We will be taking our GOAL body weight to get calculations of what our daily caloric intake SHOULD be. I used to do it with current weight but it can set some way above what's needed daily. This then leads to not seeing results & people getting discouraged because they can't reach their goals! So let's get started...

HOW MANY CALORIES TO EAT

Take your GOAL BODYWEIGHT

ex: I weigh 130lbs

WANT TO LOSE FAT?
multiply by **10-12**
ex: I would consume 1,300-1,560 calories as a starting point

WANT TO MAINTAIN?
multiply by **14**
ex: I would consume 1,820 calories as a starting point

WANT TO GAIN MUSCLE?
multiply by **16-18**
ex: I would consume 2,080-2,340 calories as a starting point

Keep in mind that these are starting points to find the total number of calories you should be eating per day to support your goals. Realistically, you need to track your calorie intake and monitor changes in bodyweight to determine if you need to be eating fewer or more calories to reach your goals at a healthy rate. Healthy fat loss happens at a rate of .5-1.5lbs/week on average

EXAMPLE:

Ellie

current weight 127

goal weight 125ish so I'm in my range

125 x 10 = 1250

125 x 12 = 1500

It's important NOT to add your workouts when tracking in apps because that will RAISE your daily caloric allowance, hence not be in a calorie deficit and wort see progress! Do your calculations & if you have questions, reach out and ask me! Contact information is at the end of the book & I'd love to help

Calculating Daily Macros Needs

This is the hard way to learn & track macros but it's a good thing to do so you see the actual numbers before I show you the much easier way with tracking apps, ratios & Portion Fix containers. Once you do this, you'll have a general idea of the basic suggested macros (carbs/fats/protein ratio) to be lean & lose, gain and/or maintain LEAN muscle mass. The numbers will help you understand your macro ratios which are easier to track than grams

I suggest having a percentage of 40-50% protein, 25-30% carbs, 30-35% fat. I've modified the math since the typical macros ratio math gives you a high carb outcome which will NOT give you the results you're looking for (leaning out/increasing lean muscle) Using a tracking app such as My Fitness PAL will help balance those percentages without having to do math daily.

Protein should be the highest, then fats and last carbs for weight loss. For maintenance and/or increasing lean muscle mass, you should still keep protein highest and can balance out carbs/fats or make one slightly higher than the other.

Remember that a calorie deficit (for weight loss) and/or meeting your daily caloric intake without going over is key for weight loss and maintenance, along with macros and the 80/20 rule. 80% clean choices & 20% not as clean. Now for the math. I recommend using your goal weight vs your current weight so you get accustomed to what you SHOULD be eating, don't over eat, hence making it easier to maintain your weight once you achieve it. See equations first then see my example below. Follow with your stats next.

STEP 1

Finding your Daily Caloric Intake

Multiply your goal weight x 10

* this is your daily caloric intake on non-workout days and/or days with less than 10K steps

* On days when you exercise for 45+ min strenuously and/or get 10K + steps in, you can raise your calories by 300 IF you're hungry & need it. But remember it's not necessary if you're not hungry, water first ALWAYS &

don't add workouts to tracking apps so it doesn't give you a false daily caloric requirement & you end up zeroing out any workouts you did by eating too much.

STEP 2

Protein Grams & Calories

Multiply your goal weight x 1.15 = Grams of protein per day

Multiply Grams of protein x 4 = Protein Calories per day

STEP 3

Fat Grams & Calories

Multiply goal weight x .35 = Grams of Fat per day

Multiply grams of fat x 9 = calorie from fat per day

STEP 4

Carbs Grams & Calories

Take your daily caloric intake and subtract your protein calories and your fat calories from it = Carb Calories for the day. Example:

Daily calories - Protein Cals - Fat Cals = Carb Cals

For carb grams per day, take your Carb calories per day divide that by 5

Macro Percentages/Ratios

Divide your calories for each macro by the total daily calories & you'll see your percentages. This is what you should adjust your macros to on your tracking app. See my example below

~~~~~~~~~~~~~~~~~~~~~~~~~~~~~~~~~~~~

Below is an example using my current body weight since I'm at my goal & maintaining::

Step 1 Multiply your goal body weight by 10.

128 x 10 = 1280

So I should consume about 1280 calories per day. If I workout 30-60 minutes per day, I can add about 300 calories so my range is about 1280-1580.

Step 2 PROTEIN

128 X 1.15 = 147 Grams of protein

x 4 = 588 protein calories

Step 3 FAT

128 x .35 = 44 grams of fat

44 x 9 = 403 fat calories

Step 4 CARBS

Total calories 1280 – protein calories (588) – fat calories (403) = 289 calories from carbs

289/ 5 = 58

Total calories per day 1280

Protein grams 147 / 588 calories ~ Fat grams 44 / 403 calories ~ Carbs grams 58 / 289 calories

Now, divide your calories for each macro by the total daily calories & you'll see your percentages. This is what you should adjust your macros to on your tracking app

Protein: 588 / 1280 = .45 (45%)

Fat: 403 / 1280 = .31 (31%)

Carbs: 289 / 1280 = .23 (23%) + 1% to = 100% (24%)

Percentages total 99 since it's approximate so add the extra 1% wherever you like. I choose carbs lol! The app (My Fitness Pal) only lets you adjust in increments of 5 so mine are set to 45% protein — 30% fats — 25% carbs

Sample Macros Ratios

Below are examples of approximate MACROS RATIOS for:

(1) Increasing Weight/Muscle

(2) Maintenance

(3) Weightloss/Fat loss

When it comes to maintenance, I choose the lower numbers for each ratio so I maintain lean mass. So I stick to about 35% protein, 30% carbs and 35% fat. When I switch back to weight loss if I see a little fluff or my weight creep up, I go to about 45% protein, 25% carbs and 30% fats. It works for me but there's a range for a reason. Some days you'll eat/indulge more than others and you just balance it out the following. It's not about perfection it's about progress & balance.. Play with the numbers in that range after tracking for a bit and see what works for you

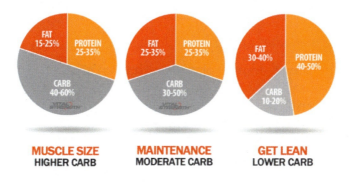

My Fitness Pal

My Fitness Pal is the tracking app I use to track my macros. When you watch the tutorial video, it walks you through how to set your goals on there so they fit your required macros ratios since the app default sets them to a high carb diet. You want to avoid that when losing weight and/or trying to gain LEAN muscle.

Once you scan in or manually add a food or meal, you will start to see your macros ratio for the day. This will change throughout the day as you eat. If you see carbs too high after breakfast for example, have a lunch higher in protein + fats. It also helps to add what you plan to eat for the day ahead of time. This is so you can see how your day will look before you begin and if you notice it's too high in one macro/too low in another, you can make changes in what you plan to eat. This also helps make room for things like dessert, cocktails, etc. If you plan on indulging in the evening, eat clean, high protein, low carb during the day & leave room for that later

Click on this LINK https://youtu.be/hJH7cglwtkA & watch the tutorial. Make sure that, before tracking, you adjust your macros (protein, fat, carbs) requirements so you aim for the right goals each day. The video shows you how to do that. Feel free to message me with questions if needed. Contact info is at the end of the book & I'm always available for questions. Then start tracking & see how tracking your macros can help you reach your goals

I'll add that tracking is VERY IMPORTANT & a NECESSARY part of understanding macros. A lot of people THINK they're eating "well, balanced, healthy" etc when in reality they're not & don't realize it until they see it by tracking. Yes it can be tedious but It's also EXTREMELY useful in learning macros & how to balance them throughout the day. EVERYTHING worthwhile in life takes work, remember that.

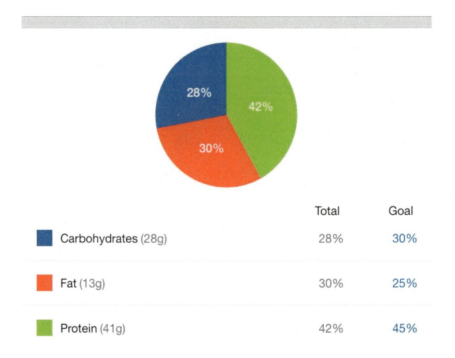

Reading Nutrition Labels

While you should always be using My Fitness Pal and tracking with it, it's also important to be able to read nutrition labels & understand what the information there means. It helps understand how many servings, calories, carbs, fats, fiber, etc you're getting in the foods you eat. Here is an example of a nutrition label with some tips on what to look for highlighted on the right

Reading Food Labels

Nutrition Facts
Serving Size 1/3 Cup (45g) Makes 1 Cup
Servings Per Container About 4

→ Start by checking the Serving Size and Servings Per Container

Amount Per Serving	Mix	As Prepared
Calories	140	210
Calories from Fat	10	15

	% Daily Value**	
Total Fat 1.5g*	2%	2%
Saturated Fat 0g	0%	0%
Trans Fat 0g		
Cholesterol 0mg	0%	0%
Sodium 850mg	35%	51%
Total Carbohydrate 22g	7%	11%
Dietary Fiber 5g	20%	40%
Sugars 5g		
Protein 12g		

→ Know labeling loopholes. If there is 0.5 g or less trans fat per serving manufacturers do not have to list it here

→ Know what you want to maximize (Fiber and protein)

→ Know what you want to minimize or avoid (sugar and sodium)

Vitamin A	10%	15%
Vitamin C	25%	40%
Calcium	6%	8%
Iron	15%	20%

*Amount in Mix. As Prepared contributes an additional 70 Calories (5 Calories from Fat), 380 mg Sodium, 12 g Total Carbohydrate (5 g Dietary Fiber, 2 g Sugars), 4 g Protein.
**Percent Daily Values are based on a 2,000 calorie diet. Your daily values may be higher or lower depending on your calorie needs:

	Calories:	2,000	2,500
Total Fat	Less than	65g	80g
Sat Fat	Less than	20g	25g
Cholesterol	Less than	300mg	300mg
Sodium	Less than	2,400mg	2,400mg
Total Carbohydrate		300g	375g
Dietary Fiber		25g	30g

INGREDIENTS (VEGAN): TEXTURED SOY PROTEIN, DEHYDRATED VEGETABLES (TOMATOES, ONIONS, GARLIC, RED BELL PEPPERS, CELERY, JALAPEÑO PEPPERS), CORN MEAL, BARLEY FLAKES, SOY SAUCE POWDER (WHEAT, SOYBEANS, SALT), SPICES, BROWN RICE SYRUP SOLIDS, SEA SALT, EXPELLER PRESSED CANOLA OIL, YEAST EXTRACT, MISO POWDER (SOYBEANS, RICE, SALT), NATURAL FLAVOR, VINEGAR POWDER, CITRIC ACID.

CONTAINS SOY AND WHEAT INGREDIENTS.
MADE ON SHARED EQUIPMENT THAT ALSO PROCESSES MILK AND PEANUTS.

→ Read the ingredients list and look out for hydrogenated and partially-hydrogenated oils, interesterified fats, high fructose corn syrup, artificial ingredients, MSG, nitrates and nitrites

→ INGREDIENTS: Textured soy protein, dehydrated vegetables (tomatoes, onions, garlic, red bell peppers, celery, jalapeño peppers), corn meal, barley flakes, soy sauce powder (wheat, soybeans, salt), spices, brown rice syrup solids, sea salt, expeller pressed canola oil, yeast extract, miso powder (soybeans, rice, salt), natural flavor, vinegar powder, citric acid.

→ Watch out for allergens!

This is the BASICS on macros & tracking them. If you'd like more information and/or help learning about macros in recipes, foods, more in depth information on creating meal plans that are macro based, contact me via email at ellieperico@aol.com or via DM on IG @fitcopmom & I'll be able to help you further.

Before going on to the Macro based meal plans, I want to address portions. The meal plans are based on approximate macro ratios for men & women BUT you also have to be careful with PORTIONS. That will make or break your results and offset your macros too if you're not being careful with them. For example, if the plan says ½ cup of rice but you have 1-2 cups (which most people have in a typical meal) it will significantly throw off your macros AND calories die the day and not see results. I discuss that further in my coaching groups with the macro Portion Fix containers.

That's where the Portion Fix program comes in. The Portion Fix program helps you put your meals together and easily get the right portions of protein, fats and carbs without needing to use a food scale. It teaches you to eyeball portions based on each macro container size so, when you're eating out or at restaurants you can easily identify what a proper portion is without needing a food scale. And who has a food scale at a restaurant with them anyway! With the containers you have 7 different colors but I condensed them to 3 to help you understand macros better.

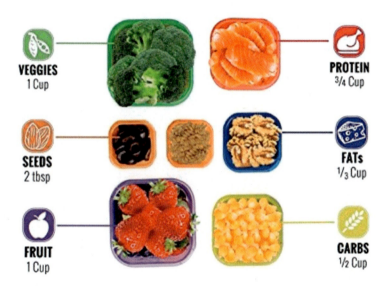

The Portion Fix containers are as follows:

Carbs = Yellow

Proteins = Red

Veggies = Green

Fruits = Purple

Healthy Fats/ Dairy = Blue

Seeds & Dressings = Orange

Oils & Nut Butters = Gray

For the purpose of learning macros, I combine them as follows:

Proteins = Red

Carbs = Yellow, Purple & Green

Fats = Blue, Orange & Gray

Proteins

Proteins are all animal proteins such as fish, poultry, beef, etc. It also includes eggs, plain Greek yogurt, cottage cheese, tofu, etc. See the red titled Protein list on page 4 of this book.

Carbs

Carbs are made up of vegetables, whole grains and all fruits. See the green and yellow list of Carbs on page 4 of this book. When it comes to carbs, some are better than others. I always encourage complex, high fiber carbs primarily in your diet. The list on page 4 shows the high fiber carbs in Green, including most vegetables & low glycemic fruits. The yellow list is the lower fiber, higher sugar carbs such as cereal, bread, tortillas, higher glycemic fruit, etc. All fruits are carbs but some are lower in sugar & higher in fiber than others. I go more in detail with this in my coaching groups & you're welcome to contact me for more information. Vegetables are a little more complicated but if you know what starchy veggies and some of the sweeter veggies are it'll help. Like I tell my clients, you want to try and fill up your plate at each meal mostly with non-starchy vegetables as often as possible. Non starchy vegetables are usually greens. Starchy vegetables are potatoes, corn, peas, squash, carrots, beets, pumpkin, plantain, squash, etc. Other sweeter veggies are sweet mini peppers, onions and tomatoes. They don't have quite as many carbs as starchy veggies but they do have some so we add them to this list. Milk is also high in sugar vs protein and it's also added to the carbs category.

Other vegetables such as leafy greens (kale, spinach, arugula) and green veggies such as cucumber, celery, etc are considered freebies in my opinion and you can load up on them! Their caloric value is so low that you can't really "overeat them" & I give myself free reign with those.

Fats

Fats include cheese, nuts, seeds, oils, salad dressings, nut butters, avocado, margarine, butter, etc. They're in the blue column in page 4.

Click this LINK https://youtu.be/K5YWyiI-qTs for more info on how the program works & this LINK https://youtu.be/aNZPHY8BRfU will help you see how I use them to assemble my meals when meal prepping. If you're interested in the program, please contact me via email (ellieperico@aol.com) or DM me on IG @fitcopmom & I'll send you a link & coach you through it FREE so you can properly learn how to use them.

Macro Meal Plan - Female - 1200 to 1600

This meal plan is for approximately 1,400 calories. If your target calorie range (or TDEE) is higher than that, you can add proteins, fats & carbs accordingly to raise the daily caloric intake & macros. It is OK if SOME days you fall below the 1,200 - 1,400 calorie range. Just try not to make it a habit so it doesn't spike cravings or leave you very hungry at the end of the day reaching for anything you see. Also, nutritional info will vary slightly in brands & sizes of foods so use My Fitness Pal to track macros & adjust serving sizes accordingly.

To raise calories add a snack & slightly increase protein servings in meals. Or you can use the Male Meal Plan & reduce some servings. You can also add ingredients to your Shakeology. If you don't have Shakeology & want some, contact me. You can use another shake but nutritional value will be different so adjust macros accordingly if they are. If you have ANY questions, ask & tag me in my Macros Support Coaching Group if you're in it. If not, email me OR contact me to join the group for additional support & 1:1 coaching. Contact info is at the end of the book.

	Breakfast	Snack	Lunch	Snack	Dinner
Monday	Spinach Avocado Egg White Omelet with Ezekiel toast	Shakeology w/ Spinach, water, ice	Lettuce wrapped Salmon burger with broccoli & quinoa	Triple Zero Vanilla Greek yogurt with almonds	Grilled Chicken breast over spring mix salad blend, tomatoes, feta cheese
Tuesday	Overnight oats or oatmeal with Greek yogurt & blueberries	Shakeology w/ Spinach, water, ice	Grilled Chicken breast over spring mix salad blend, tomatoes, feta cheese	Baby carrots and hummus String cheese & HB egg	Ground turkey breast over spaghetti squash with marinara
Wednesday	Scrambled eggs with bacon, bell peppers, mushrooms and avocado	Shakeology w/ Spinach, water, ice	Ground turkey breast over spaghetti squash with marinara	String cheese and sweet mini bell peppers	Turkey Stuffed Bell Peppers
Thursday	Egg & Oat pancakes w/ almond butter	Shakeology w/ Spinach, water, ice	Turkey Stuffed Bell Peppers	Triple Zero Vanilla Greek yogurt with almonds	Balsamic Chicken breast and Cauli Rice
Friday	Spinach Avocado Omelet with Ezekiel toast	Shakeology w/ Spinach, water, i	Balsamic Chicken Breast and Cauli Rice	Baby carrots and hummus	Salsa Chicken over Zucchini noodles and spinach
Saturday	Overnight oats with Greek yogurt & blueberries	Shakeology w/ Spinach, water, ice	Salsa Chicken over Zucchini noodles	String cheese and sweet mini bell peppers	Protein burger Beef or Turkey Breast with sweet potato fries & salad
Sunday	Scrambled eggs with bacon, bell peppers, mushrooms and avocado	Shakeology w/ Spinach, water, ice	Protein burger Beef or Turkey Breast with sweet potato fries & salad	Triple Zero Vanilla Greek yogurt with almonds	Lettuce wrapped Salmon burger with broccoli & quinoa

SPINACH AVOCADO EGG WHITE OMELET WITH EZEKIEL TOAST

8 egg whites

Handful of spinach

¼ avocado

1 slice toast

No salt seasoning of choice

1. Spray pan with non stick spray (olive oil spray is what I prefer). Pour eggs in. When bottom is well cooked, add spinach and flip top over spinach until omelet is fully cooked.
2. Serve on a plate with ¼ sliced avocado & toast

LETTUCE WRAPPED SALMON BURGER WITH QUINOA & BROCCOLI

1 Trident salmon burger patty

½ cup of cooked quinoa

1 cup steamed broccoli

1. Grill, bake or make the salmon patty on a skillet.
2. Make the quinoa as directed on package
3. Steam broccol
4. Serve together

GRILLED CHICKEN BREAST OVER SPRING MIX SALAD BLEND WITH TOMATO, BLACK OLIVES & AVOCADO

4oz chicken breast

2 cups spring mix blend

½ tomato

2 tbsp Black olives

¼ cup of feta cheese

1. Grill chicken breast, bake or make in a skillet.
2. Combine rest of ingredients in a bowl.
3. Chop chicken breast and serve over salad
4. Toss in balsamic vinegar and lime juice if desired

OVERNIGHT OATS OR OATMEAL WITH GREEK YOGURT & BLUEBERRIES

½ cup or dry oats

¾ Plain Greek yogurt or vanilla Triple Zero Oikos

1 cup blueberries

Make the oats with water as recommended in package. After it cools add in yogurt. Sprinkle cinnamon if desired and top with blueberries

GROUND TURKEY BREAST OVER SPAGHETTI SQUASH WITH MARINARA

4 oz ground turkey breast

½ cup cooked spaghetti squash

¼ cup low sugar marinara sauce

1. Place whole spaghetti squash in oven and bake for 20 min at 400
2. Remove it and cut in half.
3. Spray pan and place spaghetti squash face down. Bake for an additional 30-45 minutes
4. Set aside to cool for 15 minutes
5. Cook ground turkey in a skillet using olive oil, coconut oil ir avocado oil spray
6. Season with your choice of low sodium or no salt seasoning
7. Take a fork to the spaghetti squash and slowly pull out the "spaghetti" onto a plate
8. Add ground turkey to it, pour marinara on top and serve warm. Sprinkle Parmesan cheese on top of desired

SCRAMBLED EGGS WITH BACON, EGGS, MUSHROOM & AVOCADO

8 egg whites

2 slices of turkey bacon

1 cup mushrooms

¼ avocado

1. Cook bacon in the microwave or a pan until fully cooked.
2. Sautée mushrooms in a pan with olive oil spray.
3. Add eggs and chopped bacon
4. Scramble and cook thoroughly together
5. Serve with avocado in the side
6. Add salsa if desired

TURKEY STUFFED BELL PEPPERS

Approximate prep time: 1 hour

4 Bell Peppers (any color but red are sweetest and best choice)

1 lb. Jennie-O lean or extra lean ground turkey (plain, taco or Italian flavor)

2 cups of marinara sauce (homemade or your fave in a jar!)

1 chopped onion (optional)

1 cup rice or quinoa (optional)

2 tablespoons of garlic

1/2 cup shredded cheese or 4 slices of cheese (provolone or mozzarella)

1. Begin by rinsing and hollowing out your bell peppers. Try to use bell peppers that are large and round so they can sit well in a glass baking dish. After they're hollowed out, you can either bake them on a cookie sheet for about 20 minutes at 400 degrees to soften them up OR boil them. If you boil them, you'll need a large pot. Place them in the large pot covered in water. Bring water to a boil and let the bell peppers soften in the water for approximately 15 - 20 minutes. Once they are done, remove them from the water and place them in a square glass baking dish. For me, baking is easier :)

2. While the peppers are softening, make your rice or quinoa as you normally would. You can make it in a rice cooker or a pot. Typically it's two parts water to 1 part rice. I make 2 cups of it. Sometimes i have some left over that I just save and eat as a side dish. It's up to you how much rice/quinoa you want to add. I like mine with about 3 parts turkey to 1 part rice/quinoa.

3. As the peppers are softening and rice/quinoa is cooking, brown your onions and garlic (if you want to add them). Garlic is optional. I add garlic to almost everything but not everyone likes it in this recipe so it's up to you. If bell peppers are on sale and I buy a few extra, I also chop a bell pepper or two and brown it to add to the turkey filling along with the onions and garlic. Adds a little more substance, flavor and veggies to the recipe.

4. After browning the onions and garlic, cook the ground turkey. I place the chopped onions in a pan for a few minutes then remove them, put them aside in a bowl and cook the turkey in the same pan. Once the turkey is cooked, I add the onions and mix it together. If you buy the Jennie-O Taco or Italian turkey you won't need to add seasoning but if you buy the plain you may want to add taco seasoning to give it some flavor.

5. Once the rice/quinoa and turkey with onions is prepared, mix it together and add as much or as little of the

marinara sauce as you'd like. I typically add about 1/2 cup to a cup but I don't measure. I just go by how I like the consistency. You are now ready to stuff your peppers.

6. Stuff them with the filling. Then you can serve as is, top with more sauce and/or too with cheese & bake for an additional 5-10 minutes then remove and enjoy!

EGG WHITE & OATMEAL PROTEIN PANCAKES

1 cup egg whites

1/3 cup oats

1 packet stevia

Cinnamon to taste

****another recipe option is using Kodiak pancake mix. You can follow directions on the box OR use half Kodiak/half protein powder if desired sbd sub the water with egg whites for increased protein content

1. Spray pan with cooking spray and heat over a medium high heat
2. Stir all ingredients together until adequately combined and pour into pan
3. When the pancake begins to turn white and the edges of the pancake begin to harden, flip and cook for another one to two minutes
4. Spread nut butter if desired and enjoy

BALSAMIC VINEGAR AND CAULIFLOWER FRIED RICE

4 Oz chicken breast

Balsamic vinegar

Lime juice

1 medium-sized head of cauliflower

2 tablespoons sesame oil

1 large carrot, cubed

2 garlic cloves, minced

1 cup frozen edamame

2 beaten eggs (use scrambled tofu for vegan)

3 tablespoons low sodium soy sauce (use tamari for GF)

6 green onions, minced

***You can save time & make it easier by buying cauliflower rice already made/frozen at Costco or any grocery store.

1. Marinate chicken breast in balsamic vinegar, lemon juice, cilantro and seasoning. Barbecue it or grill it in your oven for 30 minutes or so at 400 or until it's well cooked.

2. Shred cauliflower using the largest side of a grater OR by just pulsing some rough cut pieces in a food processor; the end product should resemble smallish grains of rice.

3   Heat 1 tablespoon sesame oil in a large skillet over medium low heat. Add the carrots and garlic and stir fry until fragrant, about 5 minutes. Add the cauliflower, edamame, and remaining sesame oil to the pan; stir fry quickly to cook the cauliflower to a soft (but not mushy) texture

4   Make a well in the middle, turn the heat down, and add the eggs. Stir gently and continuously until the eggs are fully cooked. Stir in the soy sauce and green onions just before serving.

5   Serve with chicken breast

SALSA CHICKEN OVER ZUCCHINI ZOODLES AND SPINACH

4 oz chicken breasts

No salt seasoning

3 medium zucchini

2 cloves garlic, minced

2 cups packed spinach

Salt and black pepper, to taste

*** You can buy zucchini noodles already prepared at Costco or any grocery store & save time!

1. Place two chicken breasts in your slow cooker; completely cover with salsa.
2. Season as desired with no salt seasoning of your choice
3. Pour one container of salsa if your choice over the chicken. I prefer to use the chunky salsa bean and corn salsa
4. Cook on low for 3-4 hours for thawed chicken or 5-6 hours for frozen chicken
5. Once cooked, remove from heat and shred using two forks. If you are cooking for your family too,

increase the quantity of chicken breasts accordingly. You could also simply bake these in the oven, but they shred so much nicer and are so much jucier if you do it in the slow cooker.

6   Spiralize the zucchini and set aside

7   Place a large skillet over medium-high heat

8   Spray pan with olive oil spray and add the garlic, cook for 1-2 minutes

9   Add in the zucchini noodles and spinach

10 Gently toss and cook until spinach leaves are wilted, about 2-3 minutes

11 Season with no salt seasoning and freshly ground black pepper, to taste

12 Remove from heat and serve with chicken

13 Note-don't overcook the zucchini noodles and spinach or they will get soggy.

PROTEIN BURGER (LEAN BEEF or TURKEY) W/ SWEET POTATO FRIES

¼ lb 90/10 ground beef or extra lean turkey (or buy pre-made extra lean patty)

¼ onion

1 sweet potato

1. Preheat oven to 400 degrees
2. Slice sweet potato into fries of desired thickness
3. Spray cookie sheet with olive oil spray and lay sweet potato fries out
4. Spray lightly with olive oil and season with no salt seasoning and/or cinnamon
5. Bake for 25-30 minutes or until crispy
6. Remove from oven and set aside
7. Chop onion and caramelize it in a skillet using olive oil spray.
8. Blend onion into beef or turkey and form patty
9. Grill patty or make it on a skillet

Macro Meal Plan - Male - 1700 - 2,000

This meal plan is set for approximately 1,800 calories. If your target calorie range (or TDEE) is higher than that, you can add proteins, fats & carbs accordingly to raise the daily caloric intake & macros. It is OK if SOME days you fall below the 1,700 - 2,000 calorie range. Just try not to make it a habit so it doesn't spike cravings or leave you very hungry at the end of the day reaching for anything you see. Also, nutritional info will vary slightly in brands & sizes of foods so use My Fitness Pal to track macros & adjust serving sizes accordingly.

To raise calories add a snack & slightly increase protein servings in meals. Or you can use the Male Meal Plan & reduce some servings. You can also add ingredients to your Shakeology. If you don't have Shakeology & want some, contact me. You can use another shake but nutritional value will be different so adjust macros accordingly if they are. If you have ANY questions, ask & tag me in my Macros Support Coaching Group if you're in it. If not, email me OR contact me to join the group for additional support & 1:1 coaching. Contact info is at the end of the book.

	Breakfast	Snack	Lunch	Snack	Dinner
Monday	Spinach Avocado Egg White Omelet with Ezekiel toast and turkey bacon	Shakeology w/ Spinach, water, ice Carrots & Hummus	Lettuce wrapped Salmon burger with broccoli & quinoa	Triple Zero Vanilla Greek yogurt with almonds	Grilled Chicken breast over spring mix salad blend, tomatoes, feta cheese
Tuesday	Oats w/ Greek yogurt & blueberries & Ezekiel toast almond butter	Shakeology w/ Spinach, water, ice	Grilled Chicken breast over spring mix salad blend, tomatoes, feta cheese	Baby carrots and hummus String cheese & 2 HB eggs	Ground turkey breast over spaghetti squash with marinara
Wednesday	Scrambled eggs with bacon, bell peppers, mushrooms and avocado	Shakeology w/ Spinach, water, ice	Ground turkey breast over spaghetti squash with marinara	String cheese and sweet mini bell peppers Triple Zero Oikos & almonds	Turkey Stuffed Bell Peppers & Quinoa
Thursday	Egg & Oat pancakes w/ almond butter +turkey bacon	Shakeology w/ Spinach, water, ice String cheese	Turkey Stuffed Bell Peppers & quinoa	Triple Zero Vanilla Greek yogurt with almonds	Balsamic Chicken breast and Cauli Rice
Friday	Spinach Avocado Omelet Ezekiel toast	Shakeology w/ Spinach, water, ice	Balsamic Chicken Breast and Cauli Rice	Baby carrots and hummus 2 HB eggs + string cheese	Salsa Chicken over Zucchini noodles and spinach
Saturday	Overnight oats with Greek yogurt & blueberries	Shakeology w/ Spinach, water, ice	Salsa Chicken over Zucchini noodles	String cheese and sweet mini bell peppers	Protein burger Beef or Turkey Breast with sweet potato fries & salad
Sunday	Scrambled eggs with bacon, bell peppers, mushrooms and avocado	Shakeology w/ Spinach, water, ice	Protein burger Beef or Turkey Breast with sweet potato fries & salad	Triple Zero Vanilla Greek yogurt with almonds Albacore tuna & celery sticks	Lettuce wrapped Salmon burger with broccoli & quinoa

SPINACH AVOCADO EGG WHITE OMELET WITH EZEKIEL TOAST

8 egg whites

Handful of spinach

1 oz avocado

Applegate turkey bacon (2 servings)

1 slice toast

No salt seasoning of choice

1. Spray pan with non stick spray (olive oil spray is what I prefer). Pour eggs in. When bottom is well cooked, add spinach and flip top over spinach until omelet is fully cooked.

2. Serve on a plate with ¼ sliced avocado & toast

LETTUCE WRAPPED SALMON BURGER WITH QUINOA & BROCCOLI

1 Trident salmon burger patty

1 cup of cooked quinoa

1 cup steamed broccoli

1. Grill, bake or make the salmon patty on a skillet.
2. Make the quinoa as directed on package
3. Steam broccol & serve together

GRILLED CHICKEN BREAST OVER SPRING MIX SALAD BLEND WITH TOMATO & FETA CHEESE

4 oz chicken breast

2 cups spring mix blend

½ tomato

¼ cup of feta cheese

1. Grill chicken breast, bake or make in a skillet.
2. Combine rest of ingredients in a bowl.
3. Chop chicken breast and serve over salad
4. Toss in balsamic vinegar and lime juice if desired

OVERNIGHT OATS OR OATMEAL WITH GREEK YOGURT & BLUEBERRIES

½ cup or dry oats

¾ Plain Greek yogurt or vanilla Triple Zero Oikos

1 cup blueberries

1 Alice Ezekiel toast

1 Tbs almond butter

Make the oats with water as recommended in package. After it cools add in yogurt. Sprinkle cinnamon if desired and top with blueberries

GROUND TURKEY BREAST OVER SPAGHETTI SQUASH WITH MARINARA

6oz ground turkey breast

1 cup cooked spaghetti squash

¼ cup low sugar marinara sauce

1. Place while spaghetti squash in oven and bake for 20 min at 400
2. Remove it and cut in half.
3. Spray pan and place spaghetti squash face down. Bake for an additional 30-45 minutes
4. Set aside to cool for 15 minutes
5. Cook ground turkey in a skillet using olive oil non stick spray.
6. Season with your choice of low sodium or no salt seasoning
7. Take a fork to the spaghetti squash and slowly pull out the "spaghetti" onto a plate
8. Add ground turkey to it and pour marinara on top and serve warm. Sprinkle Parmesan cheese on top of desired

SCRAMBLED EGGS WITH BACON, EGGS, MUSHROOM & AVOCADO

8 egg whites

2 slices of turkey bacon

1 cup mushrooms

¼ avocado

1. Cook bacon in the microwave, air fryer or a pan until fully cooked.
2. Sautée mushrooms in a pan with olive oil spray.
3. Add eggs and chopped bacon
4. Scramble and cook thoroughly together
5. Serve with avocado in the side
6. Add salsa if desired

TURKEY STUFFED BELL PEPPERS

Approximate prep time: 1 hour

4 Bell Peppers (any color but red are sweetest and best choice)

1 lb. Jennie-O lean or extra lean ground turkey (plain, taco or Italian flavor)

2 cups of marinara sauce (homemade or your fave in a jar!)

1 chopped onion (optional)

1 cup rice or quinoa (optional)

2 tablespoons of garlic

1/2 cup shredded cheese or 4 slices of cheese (provolone or mozzarella)

1. Begin by rinsing and hollowing out your bell peppers. Try to use bell peppers that are large and round so they can sit well in a glass baking dish. After they're hollowed out, you can either bake them on a cookie sheet for about 20 minutes at 400 degrees to soften them up OR boil them. If you boil them, you'll need a large pot. Place them in the large pot covered in water. Bring water to a boil and let the bell peppers soften in the water for approximately 15 - 20 minutes. Once they are done, remove

them from the water and place them in a square glass baking dish. For me, baking is easier :)

2. While the peppers are softening, make your rice or quinoa as you normally would. You can make it in a rice cooker or a pot. Typically it's two parts water to 1 part rice. I make 2 cups of it. Sometimes i have some left over that I just save and eat as a side dish. It's up to you how much rice/quinoa you want to add. I like mine with about 3 parts turkey to 1 part rice/quinoa.

3. As the peppers are softening and rice/quinoa is cooking, brown your onions and garlic (if you want to add them). Garlic is optional. I add garlic to almost everything but not everyone likes it in this recipe so it's up to you. If bell peppers are on sale and I buy a few extra, I also chop a bell pepper or two and brown it to add to the turkey filling along with the onions and garlic. Adds a little more substance, flavor and veggies to the recipe.

4. After browning the onions and garlic, cook the ground turkey. I place the chopped onions in a pan for a few minutes then remove them, put them aside in a bowl and cook the turkey in the same pan. Once the turkey is cooked, I add the onions and mix it together. If you buy the Jennie-O Taco or Italian turkey you won't need to add seasoning but if you buy the plain you may want to add taco seasoning to give it some flavor.

5. Once the rice/quinoa and turkey with onions is prepared, mix it together and add as much or as little of the marinara sauce as you'd like. I typically add about 1/2 cup to a cup but I don't measure. I just go by how I like the consistency. You are now ready to stuff your peppers.

6. Stuff them with the filling. Then you can serve as is, top with more sauce and/or too with cheese & bake for an additional 5-10 minutes then remove and enjoy!

EGG WHITE & OATMEAL PROTEIN PANCAKES

1 cup egg whites

1/3 cup oats

1 packet stevia

1 Tbs almond butter

2 serviced Applegate turkey bacon

Cinnamon to taste

****another recipe option is using Kodiak pancake mix. You can follow directions on the box OR use half Kodiak/half protein powder if desired sbd sub the water with egg whites for increased protein content

1. Spray pan with cooking spray and heat over a medium high heat
2. Stir all ingredients together until adequately combined and pour into pan
3. When the pancake begins to turn white and the edges of the pancake begin to harden, flip and cook for another one to two minutes

BALSAMIC VINEGAR AND CAULIFLOWER FRIED RICE

6 oz chicken breast

Balsamic vinegar

Lime juice

1 medium-sized head of cauliflower

2 tablespoons sesame oil

1 large carrot, cubed

2 garlic cloves, minced

1 cup frozen edamame

2 beaten eggs (use scrambled tofu for vegan)

3 tablespoons low sodium soy sauce (use tamari for GF)

6 green onions, minced

***You can save time & make it easier by buying cauliflower rice already made/frozen at Costco or any grocery store.

1. Marinate chicken breast in balsamic vinegar, lemon juice, cilantro and seasoning. Barbecue it or grill it in your oven for 30 minutes or so at 400 or until it's well cooked.
2. Shred cauliflower using the largest side of a grater OR by just pulsing some rough cut pieces in a food

processor; the end product should resemble small-ish grains of rice.

3. Heat 1 tablespoon sesame oil in a large skillet over medium low heat. Add the carrots and garlic and stir fry until fragrant, about 5 minutes. Add the cauliflower, edamame, and remaining sesame oil to the pan; stir fry quickly to cook the cauliflower to a soft (but not mushy) texture

4. Make a well in the middle, turn the heat down, and add the eggs. Stir gently and continuously until the eggs are fully cooked. Stir in the soy sauce and green onions just before serving.

5. Serve with chicken breast

SALSA CHICKEN OVER ZUCCHINI ZOODLES AND SPINACH

6oz chicken breasts

No salt seasoning

3 medium zucchini

2 cloves garlic, minced

2 cups packed spinach

Salt and black pepper, to taste

***You can save time & make it easier by buying zucchini noodles already made/frozen at Costco or any grocery store.

1. Place two chicken breasts in your slow cooker; completely cover with salsa.
2. Season as desired with no salt seasoning of your choice
3. Pour one container of salsa if your choice over the chicken. I prefer to use the chunky salsa bean and corn salsa
4. Cook on low for 3-4 hours for thawed chicken or 5-6 hours for frozen chicken

5   Once cooked, remove from heat and shred using two forks. If you are cooking for your family too, increase the quantity of chicken breasts accordingly. You could also simply bake these in the oven, but they shred so much nicer and are so much jucier if you do it in the slow cooker.

6   Spiralize the zucchini and set aside

7   Place a large skillet over medium-high heat

8   Spray pan with olive oil spray and add the garlic, cook for 1-2 minutes

9   Add in the zucchini noodles and spinach

10 Gently toss and cook until spinach leaves are wilted, about 2-3 minutes

11 Season with no salt seasoning and freshly ground black pepper, to taste

12 Remove from heat and serve with chicken

13 Note-don't overcook the zucchini noodles and spinach or they will get soggy.

PROTEIN BURGER (LEAN BEEF or TURKEY) W/ SWEET POTATO FRIES

¼ lb 90/10 ground beef or extra lean turkey (or buy premade extra lean patty)

¼ onion

1 sweet potato

1. Preheat oven to 400 degrees
2. Slice sweet potato into fries of desired thickness
3. Spray cookie sheet with olive oil spray and lay sweet potato fries out
4. Spray lightly with olive oil and season with no salt seasoning and/or cinnamon
5. Bake for 25-30 minutes or until crispy
6. Remove from oven and set aside
7. Chop onion and caramelize it in a skillet using olive oil spray.
8. Blend onion into beef or turkey and form patty
9. Grill patty or make it on a skillet

3-7 Day Detox
*Shakeoloy optional (see below)

MEAL 1	🟨 steel-cut oats	🟥 egg whites 🥄
MEAL 2	⬜ shakelology	🟩 with spinach
MEAL 3	🟥 grilled chicken	🟨 steamed yams
MEAL 4	🟥 steamed fish	🟩 steamed veg 🥄
MEAL 5	🟥 grilled chicken	🟩 steamed veg 🥄
MEAL 6	🟥 99% ground turkey	🟩 steamed veg 🥄

🟥 3/4 Cup   🟩 1 Cup   🟨 1/2 Cup   🥄 1 tsp EV Coconut Oil

⬜ if you don't have shakeology, swap back in steamed fish, grilled chicken or lean ground turkey

3-7 Day Detox Details

1. Space your meals 2 hours apart.

2. Steamed veggie options: broccoli, asparagus, green beans, zucchini, cucumbers or bell peppers

3. Seasoning options: lemon & lime juice, vinegars, herbs and spices NO SALT!

4. Oatmeal flavorings: cinnamon, nutmeg, or 1/2 tsp of stevia

5. Drink AT LEAST one gallon of water a day - spread it out as much as possible. It will help flush out the toxins.

6. Drink extra-virgin coconut oil with meals. Microwave for 10-15 seconds to get it in liquid form.

7. Coffee or tea is ok - NO creamers or sweeteners. 1/2 tsp of stevia is ok.

8. Work out as normal. But only do this meal plan for 3 days.

3-7 Day Detox Grocery List

*this list is for 3 days. If you're doing it for 6-7 days, double the items you'll need

*egg whites are suggested if you want to substitute them for chicken, fish or turkey for any 1-2 of the meal. Fresh or frozen veggies are ok

- 1 small bottle of Extra Virgin Coconut Oil (12 tsp)
- fresh spinach
- broccoli florets*
- green beans*
- asparagus
- zucchini
- cucumbers
- bell peppers
- 3 lbs of chicken breasts (6 breasts)
- 1 lbs of white fish (3-6 filets. try to stay away from tilapia)
- 1.5 lbs of extra lean ground turkey
- 1 quart of egg whites (or 1 dozen eggs separated)
- Steel-cut oats
- 1-2 medium yams (sweet potatoes)

Best Fast Food Options

Arby's

- Roast Turkey Farmhouse Salad (no dressing)

Bojangles

- Roasted chicken bytes (no biscuit, green beans on the side)
- Grilled chicken salad (no dressing)
- Grilled Chicken sandwich (no Mayo) for lower carbs no bun or only bottom bun

Boston Market

- Turkey breast w/ steamed veggies x2 on the side
- Quarter skinless rotisserie chicke meal w/ fresh veggies on side

Burger King

- Tendergrill chicken garden salad

- Whopper junior (no mayo) no bun or half bun for lower carbs
- ⅓ Low Carb Thick Burger
- Low Carb Groled Chicken Club
- Grilled Fish Tenders + side salad

Chipotle

- Salad with lettuce, fajita veggies, any protein (chicken, sofritas or steak), pico de gallo, cheese (optional), guacamole (optional)

Chick-fil-A

- Grilled chicken sandwich extra lettuce & tomato (no bun, no mayo)
- Side salad w/ vinaigrette dressing
- Grilled Chicken Salad with Balsamic dressing
- Grilled nuggets

In n Out

- Protein style hamburger (cheese optional), no salt, no spread, mustard ok, extra lettuce & tomato

El Pollo Loco

- 2 piece meal (breast & leg) with side salad, no tortilla strips w/ balsamic dreading & steamed vegetables. Corn tortillas ok
- Grilled Skinless Meal
- Grilled chicken salad, cheese ok, no fried tortilla shell, all veggies, cheese optional
- Chicken Tortilla Soup + side of broccoli

Firehouse Subs

- Chopped salad with grilled chicken

Five Guys

- Bacon Cheeseburger, no bun, wrapped in lettuce

Hardee's

- 3 piece breaded chicken tenders

Jimmy John's

- Grilled Chicken Thigh with Caesar side salad (no dressing or croutons)
- Oven roasted Caesar wings

- Chicken breast without skin

Pizza Hut

- Backyard BBQ Chicken pizza Thin n Crispy

Popeyes

- Handcrafted blackened tenders

Panda Express

- Broccoli beer & brown rice
- Chicken w/ mushrooms & brown rice
- Stringbean chicken & brown rice
- Grilled chicken teriyaki (sauce on the side)

Panera

- Grilled teriyaki chicken
- Shanghai Angus Steak

Sonic

- Grilled chicken sandwich (no Mayo/no bun)
- Grilled chicken salad (no dressing)
- Rotisserie style chopped salad (no dressing)

Subway

- Grilled chicken salad with all of the veggies & balsamic dressing, cheese optional

Wendy's

- Power Mediterranean Chicken salad (no dressing)
- Dave's single (no bun, no Mayo)

Whataburger

- Garden salad with grilled chicken (no dressing)
- Grilled chicken sandwich (no sauce)

White Castle

- Savory Grilled Chicken Slider
- Chicken Breast slider
- Turkey Slider

Wingstop

- Plain Jumbo Wings
- Plain Chicken Tenders
- Boneless Wings (plain)

Mexican Fast Food

- Street tacos, only 1 small corn tortilla. Beef or chicken, Pico and cilantro only

Poke

- Poke bowl with seaweed, any raw fish, smelt egg ok, small portion of rice, no crab salad (imitation crab with mayo),

Any Fast Food Restaurant

- Protein style burger wrapped in lettuce, tomato, onion, pickles, no mayo, no dressing/spread but ketchup & mustard ok. Request no salt/seasoning

Thank you again for purchasing this book and trusting me to help you in your journey! I dieted my entire life & tried every "quick fix" detox, challenge, meal plan out there. I also fought sn eating disorder and battled thyroid issues for over 20 yrs. I'm off thyroid medication, beat my eating disorder, overcome emotional eating & in the best shape of my life in my 40s. I never truly saw a change in my body, energy, mood, etc until I cleaned up my diet, got control of my portions and balanced my macros. I'd love to be able to help you do the same.

Like I've said before in this book, if you have ANY QUESTIONS please don't hesitate to ask. Send me an email (ellieperico@aol.com) or a message on Instagram via my profile @fitcopmom

I also have helpful videos with recipes, nutrition tips, workouts & more on my You Tube Channel and free Facebook clean eating group where I post recipes & nutrition info as well.

If you purchased the print copy & want the links in this book sent to you, please email me or send me a message on Instagram via the contact info above

I'm always available for questions & reply typically within 24-48 hours.

Treat your body right, it's the only one you've got. You take your car for regular maintenance, make sure it has the right fuel to run right? Do the same for your body. Make yourself a priority & focus on your health!

Thank you again 🙏
Ellie B Perico

Made in the USA
Monee, IL
26 June 2024